Keto Vegetarians

Vegetarian Keto Diet Cookbook

Your Free Gifts

As a way of thanking you for the purchase, I'd like to offer you 2 complimentary gifts:

- **How To Get Through Any Weight Loss Plateau While On The Ketogenic Diet:** The title is self-explanatory; if you are struggling with getting off a weight loss plateau while on the Keto diet, you will find this free gift very eye opening on what has been ailing you. Grab your copy now by clicking/tapping here or simply enter http://bit.ly/2fantonpubketo into your browser.

- **5 Pillar Life Transformation Checklist:** This short book is about life transformation, presented in bit size pieces for easy implementation. I believe that without such a checklist, you are likely to have a hard time implementing anything in this book and any other thing you set out to do religiously and sticking to it for the long haul. It doesn't matter whether your goals relate to weight loss, relationships, personal finance, investing, personal development, improving communication in your family, your overall health, finances, improving your sex life, resolving issues in your relationship, fighting PMS successfully, investing, running a successful business, traveling etc. With a checklist like this one, you can bet that anything you do will seem a lot easier to implement until the end. Therefore, even if you don't continue reading this book, at least read the one thing that will help you in every other aspect of your life. Grab your copy now by clicking/tapping here or simply enter http://bit.ly/2fantonfreebie into your browser. Your life will never be the same again (if you implement what's in this book), I promise.

PS: I'd like your feedback. If you are happy with this book, please leave a review on Amazon.

Introduction

The Ketogenic diet is undoubtedly the most effective weight loss diet, which brings sustainable fast results, as it turns the body into an efficient fat burning machine. But as you are well aware, animal products like meats form a huge part of the diet. This essentially means if you cannot eat meat e.g. if you are a vegetarian, it can be very hard to follow the diet since many of the recipes available online mainly focus on meat laden Keto.

The question you might be having right now is; so does that mean you cannot be on the Ketogenic diet if you are vegetarian? And the answer is simple; absolutely not.

You can follow the Ketogenic diet comfortably even if you are a vegetarian and this book will show you exactly how to go about following the Ketogenic diet as a vegetarian.

Let's begin.

I hope you enjoy it!

Table of Contents

Your Free Gifts ---------------------------------- 2

Introduction ------------------------------------- 4

Breakfast Recipes ------------------------------- 12

Cinnamon Faux Cereal ---------------------------- 12

Keto Porridge ------------------------------------ 14

Cinnamon Keto Granola --------------------------- 17

Chia Pudding ------------------------------------- 19

Green Coffee Shake ------------------------------- 21

Low Carb Vegan Pancakes ------------------------- 22

Keto Deviled Eggs -------------------------------- 24

Eggs in Avocado ---------------------------------- 26

Keto Cheese Omelet ------------------------------- 28

Shakshuka -- 30

Keto Main Meals --------------------------------- 33

Keto Cauliflower Mac And Cheese ----------------- 33

Crust-Less Spinach Cheese Pie -------------------- 35

Caviar Crepes ------------------------------------ 36

Keto Cheese Taco Shells -------------------------- 38

Zucchini Noodles with Avocado Sauce ------------- 40

Keto Cauliflower Mashed -------------------------- 42

Courgette Mint and Feta Fritters ----------------- 44

Pan Roasted Portobello Egg ---------------------- 45
Keto Grilled Cheese Sandwich -------------------- 47
Eggplant Parmesan Bites ------------------------ 49
Cheesy Cauliflower Casserole -------------------- 51
Broccoli Cheese Soup --------------------------- 53

Keto Desserts ------------------------------------- 55
Coconut Snowball Cookies ----------------------- 55
Peanut Butter Protein Bars ---------------------- 57
Keto Ice Cream -------------------------------- 59
Low Carb Dairy Free Fondue -------------------- 60
Keto Chocolate Truffle -------------------------- 62
Chocolate Hazelnut Cookies --------------------- 64
Chocolate Blueberry Clusters -------------------- 66
Avocado Chocolate Mousse ---------------------- 68
Strawberry Cheesecake Salad -------------------- 70

Keto Snacks and Smoothies ------------------ 72
Parmesan Cauliflower Steak --------------------- 74
Garlic Baked Brie Recipe ------------------------ 76
Baked Cheddar Parmesan Crisps ------------------ 77
Creamed Leeks with Garlic and Cream Cheese 79
Creamy Mushroom and Cauliflower Risotto --- 80
Arugula Strawberry Salad ----------------------- 82
Creamy Keto Smoothie -------------------------- 84

Coconut Vanilla Smoothie ------------------------- *86*
Low Carb Strawberry Smoothie ----------------- *87*
Chocolate Coconut Smoothie -------------------- *88*
Coconut Bacon ---------------------------------- *90*
Lemon & Garlic Sautéed Brussels sprouts ------- *92*
Stuffed Baby Peppers -------------------------------- *94*
Keto Kale Chips -------------------------------------- *95*
Creamy Cucumber Salad ---------------------------- *96*
Avocado Salad -- *97*
Avocado, Almond & Blueberry Salad ------------- *98*
Brussels Sprouts Caesar Salad --------------------- *99*
Feta Lemon Coleslaw ----------------------------- *100*
Lemon & Feta Summer Zucchini Salad -------- *102*
Tofu Fries -------------------------------------- *104*
Tempeh Stir-Fry ------------------------------- *106*
Keto Smoked Maple Tempeh ------------------- *108*
Tempeh Hash Browns ------------------------------ *110*
Spinach Almond Stir-Fry ------------------------ *111*
Green Spinach Smoothie -------------------------- *112*

Conclusion ------------------------------------- **113**

Do You Like My Book & Approach To Publishing? ------------------------------------- **114**

1: First, I'd Love It If You Leave a Review of This Book on Amazon. --------------------------------- 114

2: Check Out My Other Keto Diet Books ------- 114

3: Let's Get In Touch ----------------------------- 116

4: Grab Some Freebies On Your Way Out; Giving Is Receiving, Right? ------------------------------- 116

5: Suggest Topics That You'd Love Me To Cover To Increase Your Knowledge Bank --------------- 117

PSS: Let Me Also Help You Save Some Money! --- 118

Copyright 2018 by Fantonpublishers.com - All rights reserved.

PS:

I have special interest in the Ketogenic diet. My wife has been following the Ketogenic diet and I can honestly say that the journey has been amazing. The diet works. And this is why I have committed to writing and publishing as many of the Ketogenic diet books as possible to give readers different options as far as the Ketogenic diet is concerned.

For instance, I have Ketogenic diet books exclusively dedicated for:

- Breakfast
- Main Meals
- Snacks
- Desserts
- Appetizers
- Soups
- Vegetarians
- Crockpot/slow cooker users
- Instant pot users
- Air fryer users
- People who are on the Paleo diet
- People who are following intermittent fasting

- People who are following carb cycling

And much more.

You can check out my [Ketogenic Diet Books fan page shop](#) for more of the books, as I continue publishing more and more. If you want me to add your category of the Ketogenic diet books that I have published so far, make sure to send me a message. I will do the heavy lifting for you and get back to you with a book that you will love.

You could also subscribe to my newsletter to receive updates whenever I have something new: http://bit.ly/2Cketodietfanton.

Breakfast Recipes

Cinnamon Faux Cereal

Prep time: 5 minutes

Cook time: 25 minutes

Total time: 30 minutes

Yields: 6 (1/2 cup servings)

Ingredients

1 tablespoon of coconut oil

1/2 cup of apple cider

2 tablespoons of ground cinnamon

1/2 cup of hulled hemp seeds

1/2 cup of milled flax seed

Directions

Preheat the oven to 300 degrees F.

Mix all dry ingredients in a food processor, blender or magic bullet. Add the coconut oil and apple cider and process until the ingredients are mostly smooth and fully combined.

Spread the batter on a cookie sheet lined with parchment until nice and thin – about 1/16th inch thick

Bake in the preheated oven for 15 minutes then lower the heat to 250 degrees and bake for 10 more minutes

Remove from oven and cut into squares using a knife or a pizza cutter to about the size of the keys in a computer keyboard

Switch off the oven and place the cereal back in the oven until it is completely dried out and crisp.

Serve with coconut milk or unsweetened almond milk.

Nutritional info: Calories 129, Protein 9g, Carbs 1.25g and Fat 9g

Keto Porridge

Prep time: 5 minutes

Cook time: 20 minutes

Total time: 30 minutes

Yields: 1 serving

Ingredients

1 ½ cups of unsweetened almond milk

2 tablespoons of vegan vanilla protein powder

3 tablespoons of golden flaxseed meal

2 tablespoons of coconut flour

Powdered erythritol to taste

Directions

Mix the protein powder, golden flaxseed meal and coconut flour in a bowl

Place the above mixture in a saucepan and add the almond milk then cook over medium heat; will appear very loose at first.

Stir in your preferred amount of sweetener once it thickens

Serve with your favorite toppings

Nutritional info: Calories 249, Protein17.82g, Carbs 5.78g and Fats 13.07g

Keto Bread Recipe (For Making The Above French Toast)

Prep time: 10 minutes

Cook time: 30 minutes

Total time: 40 minutes

Yields: 20 slices

Ingredients

3 teaspoons of baking powder

4 tablespoons of melted butter

1 ½ cup of almond flour

1 pinch of pink salt

6 large eggs, separated

½ cup almond flour

Optional: ¼ teaspoon of cream of tartar

Optional: 6 drops liquid stevia

Directions

Preheat your oven to 375 degrees F.

Separate the egg yolks from the egg whites. Add cream of tartar to the egg whites and beat until you achieve soft peaks.

Add the melted butter, egg yolks, baking powder, almond flour, salt and 1/3 of the beaten egg whites to the food processor and mix until combined (adding the liquid stevia to the batter helps in reducing the mild egg taste). The resulting mixture will be thick lumpy dough until you add the remaining egg whites

Add the rest of the egg whites and process gently until fully incorporated. Ensure you do not over mix the ingredients, as the resulting mixture is what gives the bread its volume

Oil an 8x4- inch loaf pan and pour in the mixture. Place in oven and bake for 30 minutes. To ensure the bread is cooked through, check by inserting a toothpick

Nutritional info: Calories 90, Protein 3g, Carbs 2g and Fats 7g

Cinnamon Keto Granola

Prep time: 5 minutes

Cook time: 20 minutes

Total time: 25 minutes

Yields: 4 servings

Ingredients

4 tablespoons of sugar free maple syrup

1.5 oz. nuts (this recipe used almonds, walnuts and pecans)

1 tablespoon of chia seeds

5 tablespoons of unsweetened coconut flakes

5 tablespoons of ground flax meal

Optional: 1 ½ teaspoons of ground cinnamon

Directions

Combine all ingredients apart from the cinnamon.

Spread the mixture out onto a baking sheet to form a single layer.

Sprinkle the cinnamon on top of the mixture.

Bake for 20-22 minutes in the oven at 350 degrees

Let it rest, as the granola will harden when it cools. Enjoy

Nutritional info: Calories 175, Protein 6g, Carbs 11g and Fats 17g

Chia Pudding

Prep time: 0 minutes

Cook time: 20-30 minutes

Total time: 30 minutes

Yields: 1 serving

Ingredients

1 tablespoon alcohol free orange extract

2-3 tablespoons chia seeds

1 cup unsweetened coconut milk

To make the recipe even tastier there are a couple of additional ingredients that you may consider adding e.g. Blackberries, strawberries, blueberries, cocoa nibs, protein powder, MCT oil, any keto-approved sweetener you like, nuts and nut butters.

Directions

Place all ingredients plus any of your desired additional ingredients mentioned above in a bowl or 16 oz. Mason jar. If you are using the jar put the lid on tight, shake and leave to rest for 20-30 minutes or leave in fridge overnight. If using the bowl, mix all ingredients and the additional ones and let it sit for the above mentioned time.

Your pudding can be anywhere from firm to slightly runny depending on your preference.

Nutritional info: Calories 165, Protein 6g, Carbs 1g and Fat 10.5g

Green Coffee Shake

Prep time: 5 minutes

Cook time: 0

Total time: 5 minutes

Yields: 4 servings

Ingredients

2 tablespoons of unsweetened almond butter

1 1/2 cup of chilled brewed coffee (regular or decaf)

1 13.5 fl. oz. (400 ml) can of full-fat coconut milk

8 ice cubes, for serving

Directions

Add all ingredients apart from the ice cubes to your blender and blend until smooth for around 10 seconds.

Divide the shake among four 300 ml (10 fl. Oz.) glasses and drop 2 ice cubes in each glass

Enjoy!

Nutritional info: Calories 262, Protein 4.1g, Carbs 4.4g and Fat 24.9g

Low Carb Vegan Pancakes

Prep time: 5 minutes

Cook time: 10 minutes

Total time: 20 minutes

Yields: 1 batch of pancakes

Ingredients

1/2 teaspoon of baking powder

1 tablespoon of coconut flour

1 tablespoon of ground flax

1/4 cup of unsweetened almond milk

2 tablespoons of unsweetened almond butter

Optional: swerve or liquid stevia to taste

*if not using salted almond butter add a pinch of salt to your ingredients

Directions

Heat your frying pan or iron skillet over low-medium heat and lightly oil the pan with the oil of your choice.

Combine the almond milk and almond butter in a small dish and in another combine the dry ingredients until they are well mixed.

Combine the dry and wet ingredients and stir until they are thoroughly mixed. Leave the mixture to sit for a minute or two so that the coconut flour and the flax can absorb the liquid.

Spoon the batter onto your frying pan or skillet and spread gently to form pancakes. If your batter is a bit difficult to spread, you can wet the back of a spoon and use it as a spatula.

Cook until the pancake flips easily – around 4-5 minutes however check it at the third minute by shimmying the spatula under the pancake gently. (You want to see little bubbles all over the pancake surface just like in conventional pancakes.)

When the underside turns golden, flip and cook for 2-3 more minutes until done

Top with more almond butter, berries, sugar free syrup, coconut cream or vegan butter (or any combination of the foods mentioned above) and enjoy.

Nutritional info per serving: Calories 260, Protein 9.6g, Carbs 5.1 g Fat 20.8g

Keto Deviled Eggs

Prep time: 10 minutes

Cook time: 15 minutes

Total time: 25 minutes

Yields: 6 servings

Ingredients

½ tablespoon poppy seeds

¼ teaspoon salt

½ cup mayonnaise

½ avocado

1 teaspoon lime juice

6 eggs

Directions

Place the eggs in a pan and add just enough cold water to cover the eggs. Without covering with a lid, bring to a boil.

Allow the eggs to simmer in the hot water for about eight minutes then quickly cool in ice-cold water.

Carefully remove the eggshells. Cut off both ends then slice the egg into equal halves. Remove the egg yolk and place in a separate small bowl.

Place the egg whites on another plate and leave to sit in the refrigerator.

Mix the egg yolks, mayonnaise, avocado and lime juice into a smooth batter. Add salt to taste.

Take the egg whites out of the refrigerator and put the avocado mixture the place where the yolk was.

Sprinkle the poppy seeds on top and serve.

Nutritional information per 2-piece serving: Calories 200, Protein 6g, Carbs 1g and Fats 19g

Eggs in Avocado

Prep time: 5 minutes

Cook time: 25 minutes

Total time: 30 minutes

Yields: 2 boats

Ingredients

2 organic, free-range eggs

1 large ripe avocado

1 teaspoon coconut oil

Salt and pepper to taste

Garnish:

Balsamic pearls (or balsamic reduction)

Fresh thyme

Few pieces of walnuts, chopped

Directions

Slice the avocado in half then remove the pit and scoop out some flesh in order to fit an entire egg inside.

Remove a small piece of the avocado skin at the back so that it can sit straight when you place it on the cutting board.

Crack the eggs and divide them among three containers. Place the yolks in small teacups or individual shot glasses then place the egg whites together in the same mixing bowl - small in size. Add pepper and salt to the whites to taste and mix them well

Add the coconut oil to a skillet with a fitting lid and heat over medium high heat. Add the avocado halves with the flesh side down and sear until slightly golden for around 30 seconds

Flip over the avocados and fill the cavities with the egg whites almost to the top. Turn down the heat and place the lid on skillet then cook for around 15 – 20 minutes until the egg whites are about to fully set.

Slide the yolks over the egg whites carefully and cook until the yolks reach your desired level of doneness for around 3-5 minutes

Place on a serving plate and garnish with balsamic pearls, thyme and walnuts

Nutritional info (serving size 130g): Calories 215, Protein 9.1g, Carbs 8g and Fats 18.1g

Keto Cheese Omelet

Prep time: 5 minutes

Cook time: 10 minutes

Total time: 15 minutes

Yields: 2 servings

Ingredients

7 oz. cheddar cheese, shredded

6 eggs

3 oz. butter

Salt and pepper to taste

Directions

Whisk the eggs until slightly frothy and smooth. Blend half of the shredded cheese into the eggs. Add salt and pepper to taste.

In a hot frying pan, melt the butter. Add in the cheesy egg mixture and leave to sit for a few minutes.

Lower the heat and keep cooking the egg mixture until it is almost cooked through.

Add the rest of the shredded cheddar cheese, fold and serve immediately

Nutritional info: Calories 214, Protein 40g, Carbs 4g and Fats 80g

Shakshuka

Prep time: 10 minutes

Cook time: 10 minutes

Total time: 20 minutes

Yields: 1 serving

Ingredients

1/8 teaspoon of cumin

1 oz. of feta cheese

4 eggs

1 chili pepper

1 cup of marinara sauce (see recipe below)

Pepper to taste

Fresh basil

Salt to taste

Directions

Preheat oven to 400 degrees F.

Add a cup of marinara sauce and chopped chili pepper to a small skillet and heat on a medium flame. Let the chili pepper cook in the sauce for about 5 minutes.

Crack the eggs and gently pour them into the marinara sauce.

Sprinkle the eggs with feta cheese then season with cumin, pepper and salt.

Place the skillet in the oven and bake for about 10 minutes.

Remove the skillet from the oven using an oven mitt once the eggs are cooked but are still runny.

Sprinkle some fresh chopped basil over the shakshuka and enjoy

Nutritional info: Calories 490, Protein 35g, Carbs 4g and Fat 34g

Keto Marinara Sauce (For Use In Making The Above Shakshuka Recipe)

Prep time: 10 minutes

Cook time: 20 minutes

Total time: 30 minutes

Yields: 8 servings

Ingredients

5g of Fresh or dried oregano

1 tablespoon of butter

2 tablespoons of olive oil

5g of chopped garlic

50g of diced red onion

400g tomatoes (fresh or pureed)

Handful of freshly chopped basil and chili flakes

Directions

Heat the olive oil in a saucepan then add the chopped onion and season with salt. Fry until translucent.

Add in the chili flakes and the chopped onion and cook until they turn golden brown. Add the tomatoes and season with pepper and salt.

Cover and leave to cook until the oil separates from the tomatoes for around 10-12 minutes.

Add the basil and fresh oregano and cook for 2 to 3 more minutes.

Finish by adding a tablespoon of butter.

Nutritional info per serving: Calories 71, Protein 1g, Carbs 2g and Fats 7g

Keto Main Meals

Keto Cauliflower Mac And Cheese

Preparation time: 5 minutes

Cook time: 15 minutes

Total time: 20 minutes

Yields: 4 – 1 cup servings

Ingredients

¼ cup of unsweetened almond milk (or any milk of your choice)

¼ cup of heavy cream

1 cup of cheddar cheese (shredded)

3 tablespoons of butter (split into 2 tablespoons and 1 tablespoon)

1 head cauliflower (cut into little florets)

Salt and pepper to taste

Directions

Preheat your oven to 232 degrees C (450 degrees F). Use a parchment paper or foil to line a baking sheet.

Melt 2 tablespoons of butter. Toss together the melted butter with the cauliflower florets in a large bowl. Season with black pepper and salt.

Arrange the butter tossed cauliflower florets on to the lined baking sheet and roast until crisp-tender for about 10-15 minutes.

Heat the remaining tablespoon of butter, milk, heavy cream and cheddar cheese stirring frequently – you can do this in the microwave or on the stove in the double broiler. Heat your cheese mixture until it becomes smooth but ensure you are careful enough not to burn the cheese or overheat it.

Right before serving, toss the cauliflower with the cheese sauce.

Enjoy

Nutritional info per serving: Calories 294, Protein 11g, Carbs 12g and Fats 23g

Crust-Less Spinach Cheese Pie

Prep time: 2 minutes

Cook time: 25-30 minutes

Total time: 30 minutes

Yields: 8 slices

Ingredients

¼ teaspoon of garlic powder

1 teaspoon of dried minced onion

2 ½ cups of any cheese – your preferred kind

5 eggs, beaten

10 ounces of wilted down fresh spinach (or use frozen, thawed, squeezed and drained spinach)

Salt and pepper to taste

Directions

Start by greasing a 9-inch pie pan then proceed to mix all the ingredients and pour them onto the pan that you just greased. Bake at 375 degrees F for about 30 minutes or until the edges start to brown.

Nutritional info per serving: Calories 190, Protein 13.3g, Carbs 2.1g and Fats 14.6g

Caviar Crepes

Prep time: 10 minutes

Cook time: 10 minutes

Total time: 20 minutes

Yields: 2 servings

Ingredients

Blini

½ teaspoon of baking powder

2 large eggs

2 oz. cream cheese

1 pinch of sea salt

Filling

¾ cup of caviar

½ cup of sour cream

Directions

Combine all the ingredients in a blender or food processor and blend until smooth to prepare the blini style crepes.

Add a bit of butter to a small skillet and heat up over medium heat. Allow it to fully heat up. Ladle a less than ¼ cup of batter at a time then swirl the skillet in order to spread the contents around evenly.

Allow to cook until the edges begin to peel off the skillet and the bubbles have already formed on top. This should take around 2 or 3 minutes per crepe.

Flip and leave to cook for one more minute. Repeat this process with the rest of the batter.

(This recipe should yield 4 medium sized crepes). Once the crepes are ready and the batter has cooked, spoon 2 tablespoons of the sour cream onto every crepe then proceed to add 2 -3 tablespoons of the caviar and roll them up

Enjoy.

Nutritional info: Calories 535, Fat 38g, Protein 40g, Net Carbs 4g

Keto Cheese Taco Shells

Prep time: 10 minutes

Cook time: 5 minutes

Total time: 15 minutes

Yields: 6 servings

Ingredients

1/8 teaspoon of chili powder

¼ teaspoon of cumin

2 cups of shredded cheddar cheese

Directions

Preheat your oven to 191 degrees C (375 degrees F). Line either one XL baking sheet or two jelly roll pans with parchment paper.

On the baking sheet(s), place the cheese in circles with even thickness throughout then sprinkle with chili powder and cumin

Bake until bubbles start to form and the edges begin to brown for around 5-7 minutes. Meanwhile, across 2 overturned glasses, set up wooden spoons sitting horizontally. This way they are ready when you take out the cheese taco shells from the oven when they are done cooking.

Remove the pan (s) from the oven and leave to cool without disturbing for around a minute.

Use a spatula or flat turner to lift the cooked cheese circles and place them over the wooden spoon. Allow them to hang for about 5 minutes until hardened

Nutritional info per serving: Calories 152, Protein 9g, Carbs 0.4g and Fats 12g

Zucchini Noodles with Avocado Sauce

Prep time: 10 minutes

Cook time: 10 minutes

Total time: 20 minutes

Yields: 2 servings

Ingredients

12 sliced cherry tomatoes

1 avocado

2 tablespoons of lemon juice

4 tablespoons of pine nuts

1 zucchini

1 ¼ cup of basil

1/3 cup of water

Directions

Use the Spiralizer or a peeler to make the zucchini noodles.

Place all the other ingredients apart from the cherry tomatoes into a blender and blend until smooth.

Mix the cherry tomatoes, blended avocado sauce and the noodles in a mixing bowl.

*This is best eaten fresh but you can also store in the fridge for 1 to 2 days.

Nutritional info per serving: Calories 313, Protein 6.8g, Carbs 9g and Fats 26.8g

Keto Cauliflower Mashed

Prep time: 5 minutes

Cook time: 10 minutes

Total time 15 minutes

Yields: 4 servings

Ingredients

1 tablespoon of chopped chives

1 tablespoon of full fat coconut milk

3 tablespoons of olive oil

3 cloves of garlic, minced

1 head cauliflower (with the stems removed – florets only)

¾ teaspoon of sea salt

1/8 teaspoon of black pepper to taste - adjustable

Directions

Cook the cauliflower in the microwave or on the stove.

Microwave method: In a large bowl place the cauliflower florets and 2 tablespoons of water. Cover with plastic wrap and ensure it does not touch the cauliflower. Microwave for about 10 minutes on high until very soft, ensuring you stir half way through. Drain well

Stove method: Bring a pot of water with a tablespoon of salt to a boil then add the cauliflower. Simmer for about 5-6 minutes until very soft. Drain well.

Meanwhile, place the milk/cream, olive oil and garlic in a high power blender or food processor

*If you want to mellow the garlic flavor a bit, you can sauté the garlic first.

Drain well once the cauliflower is done cooking. Squeeze out the extra water by pressing a bowl down on the cauliflower over a strainer or by wrapping it in a towel then twisting

Add the cauliflower to the blender or food processor and process until smooth while scraping down on the sides occasionally with a spatula

Add the pepper and salt to taste and puree once again

You can thin out the mixture with more cream/milk if it is thicker than you like

Stir in the chopped chives

Nutritional info: Calories 139, Protein 4g, Carbs 5g and Fats 10g

Courgette Mint and Feta Fritters

Prep time: 5 minutes

Cook time: 10 minutes

Total time: 15 minutes

Yields: 4 servings

Ingredients

2 medium eggs

1 handful of fresh mint, chopped roughly

50g of feta cut into cubes

5 medium zucchini/courgettes, shredded/grated

Butter or coconut oil for frying

Directions

Grate the zucchini/courgette and squeeze out as much water as possible.

Add the eggs, feta and mint then stir through.

Heat a frying pan with butter or coconut oil, add the mixture in small batches and cook until golden.

*Depending on how large your zucchinis are, you may need to add extra eggs to hold the fritters together

Nutritional info per serving: Calories 80, Protein 5.5g, Carbs 4g and Fats 4.5g

Pan Roasted Portobello Egg

Prep time: 25 minutes

Cook time: 25 minutes

Total time: 50 minutes

Yields: 4 servings

Ingredients

6-8 cloves of garlic

4 medium/small tomatoes

2 Portobello mushrooms

Olive oil for cooking

4 eggs

Salt and pepper to taste

Garnishing: fresh thyme

Directions

Halve the Portobello mushrooms.

Pour the olive oil in a large frying pan then add the mushrooms and cook over medium heat for about 10 minutes on the stove until kind of crispy on the edges and soft on the other parts (5 minutes each side). Set the mushrooms aside once done cooking.

Slice the tomatoes in half and cook in the frying pan drizzled with enough olive oil to avoid burning or sticking. Cook for around 5 minutes – 10 minutes on each side. Remove the tomatoes from the pan once they are done cooking and set aside.

Mince the garlic then sauté in a pan drizzled with olive oil until crispy and golden for about a minute then set aside.

Fry the eggs as desired then assemble the mushroom "toast" and finally top with the fresh thyme leaves, crispy garlic, fresh cracked pepper and sea salt

Nutritional info: Calories 162, Protein 8g, Carbs 8g and Fats 12g

Keto Grilled Cheese Sandwich

Prep time: 1 min

Cook time: 2 min

Total time: 3 minutes

Yields: 1 serving

Ingredients

½ teaspoon of baking powder

1 ½ tablespoons of psyllium husk powder

2 tablespoons of almond flour

2 large eggs

3 tablespoons of soft butter

Fillings and extras

2 ounces of cheddar cheese

Directions

Place 2 tablespoons of butter in a mug and let it come to room temperature. Once it is soft, add the baking powder, psyllium husk and almond flour. Mix thoroughly in order to form thick dough.

Crack the eggs, pour into the mixture and keep mixing. The dough should be pretty thick so if yours isn't, keep mixing because it thickens more as you mix – this can go for as long as 60 seconds

Pour the dough into a bowl or square container, level it off as best as you can and clean off the sides so that it comes out as leveled as you can get it.

Microwave for around 90 to 100 seconds but check on the doneness to ensure it does not need longer.

Remove from the bowl or container by flipping it upside down and tapping the bottom lightly. Use a bread knife to cut it in half.

Measure out the amount of cheese you can fit in between the buns.

Heat 1 tablespoon of butter in a pan over medium heat. Add the buns once the butter is hot and leave to cook. The bread should absorb the butter as you cook and have a delicious crisp outside.

You can serve up with a side salad if desired

Nutritional info: Calories 803, Protein 25.84g, Carbs 6.14g and Fats 69.95g

Eggplant Parmesan Bites

Prep time: 10 minutes

Cook time: 15 minutes

Total time: 25 minutes

Yields: 2 servings

Ingredients

1 egg, lightly beaten

Salt and pepper to taste

1 eggplant/aubergine, sliced

Herb and cheese crust:

1 tablespoon of dried herbs of your choice

25 g almond flour/meal

50 and 25 grams of shredded/grated cheese of your choice

Directions

Oil your baking tray and place the sliced eggplants on top then sprinkle each slice with pepper and salt.

Grill on medium or bake at 350 degrees F/180 degrees C until browned.

As the eggplants are grilling or baking, mix all ingredients of the herb and cheese crust in a small bowl.

Remove the eggplants from the oven then flip them over and sprinkle with more pepper and salt.

Place back in the oven and grill until just cooked and turning brown – if cooked for too long the eggplant can easily become incredibly soft thus more difficult to hold so they should be slightly firm.

Remove the cooked eggplant slices from the oven then brush with the beaten egg.

Sprinkle the top with the herb and cheese crust and place back in grill/oven to cook until the cheese is just melted and is starting to brown.

Serve with garlic mayonnaise, salted yoghurt or sour cream as a side sauce

Nutritional info per serving: Calories 72, Proteins 3.9g, Carbs 2.6g and Fats 4.5g

Cheesy Cauliflower Casserole

Prep time: 10 minutes

Cook time: 15 minutes

Total time: 25 minutes

Yields: 6 servings

Ingredients

1 teaspoon of garlic powder

2 cups of cheddar cheese, shredded and divided

2 teaspoons of Dijon mustard

2 oz. cream cheese

1 cup heavy cream

1 whole cauliflowerhead, cut into florets

Salt and pepper to taste

Directions

Preheat your oven to 375 degrees F. Grease a 9x9 baking dish.

Add water to a large pot and bring to boil. Add in the cauliflower florets and half a teaspoon of salt. Leave to cook until the cauliflower is just tender - ensure you don't overcook

Drain the cooked cauliflower well then place back in the pot and set aside.

Add the cream to a small saucepan and bring to a simmer, ensuring you stir well to avoid scorching. Whisk in the mustard and the cream cheese then stir until the mixture thickens

Remove from heat and whisk in the seasonings and a cup of shredded cheese. Pour the cauliflower over and mix gently to combine.

Place the cauliflower in the dish you had prepared earlier and sprinkle the remaining cheese. Bake for about 15 minutes until the cheese is slightly browned and bubbly.

If you want an extra bubby topping, leave to broil for 2 to 3 minutes on high but ensure you watch it carefully so that it doesn't burn

Nutritional information per serving: Calories 362, Proteins 13g, Carbs 4g and Fats 33g

Broccoli Cheese Soup

Prep time: 5 minutes

Cook time: 20 minutes

Total time: 25 minutes

Yields: 8 servings

Ingredients

3 cups of pre shredded cheddar cheese

1 cup of heavy cream

3 ½ cups of vegetable stock

4 cloves of garlic, minced

4 cups of broccoli, cut into florets

Directions

Sauté the garlic in a large pot over medium heat for about a minute or until fragrant.

Add the chopped broccoli, heavy cream and vegetable stock then increase the heat and bring to boil. Reduce the heat and simmer until the broccoli is tender; around 10 to 20 minutes

Gradually add the shredded cheddar cheese stirring constantly and keep stirring until melted (add ½ a cup and simmer then stir until it fully melts then keep adding ½ cup at a time until you use up all the cheese). Ensure you avoid high heat and keep it to a very low simmer to prevent seizing.

Once all the cheese melts remove from heat immediately

Nutritional info per serving: Calories 291, Proteins 13g, Carbs 5g and Fats 25g

Keto Desserts

Coconut Snowball Cookies

Prep time: 1 minute

Cook time: 4 minutes

Total time: 5 minutes

Yields: 40 cookies

Ingredients

½ cup of coconut milk or any other milk of your choice

¼ cup of granulated sweetener of your choice

4 cups of unsweetened coconut, shredded

Optional:

¼ teaspoon of almond or vanilla extract

Directions

In a high-speed food processor or blender, add the unsweetened coconut and blend to a fine texture for 1 to 2 minutes. Do not overblend as you will end up with coconut butter

Add the coconut milk, granulated sweetener and the almond/vanilla extract if using, then blend to form a sticky thick batter. Add a little extra milk of your choosing if the batter is too crumbly

Transfer the batter onto a large mixing bowl. Wet your hands lightly then shape the batter into small balls. Place the balls onto a lined plate or baking tray.

Press the batter balls into a cookie shape and sprinkle with extra granulated sweetener or coconut.

Refrigerate until they firm up slightly.

*You can keep the cookies at room temperature, covered. They are also freezer friendly

Nutritional info: Calories 40, Proteins 1g, Carbs 2g and Fats 4g

Peanut Butter Protein Bars

Prep time: 5 minutes

Cook time: 5 minutes

Total time: 10 minutes

Yields: 24 bars

Ingredients

½ cup of sticky sweetener of your choice

2 cups of peanut butter

2 scoops of protein powder of your choice

½ cup of coconut flour

Optional:

2 cups of chocolate chips

Directions

Prepare a deep pan by lining with parchment paper and put aside. If you want thicker bars, use an 8 x 8-inch pan. If you want thinner bars, use any size bigger.

Add the dry ingredients to a large mixing bowl and mix well.

Melt the peanut butter with the sticky sweetener in a small mixing bowl until combined. Add the peanut butter mixture to the dry ingredients mixture and mix until fully combined

Transfer the batter onto the earlier prepared baking dish and press them firmly into place. Refrigerate or freeze until firm then cut into squares.

Cover in chocolate (optional) and enjoy.

*To keep the bars sugar free and keto, use a monk fruit Maple syrup

Nutritional info: Calories 139, Proteins 8g, Carbs 6g and Fats 10g

Keto Ice Cream

Prep time: 10 minutes

Cook time: 0 minutes

Total time: 10 minutes

Yields: 4-5 servings

Ingredients

1 ½ teaspoons of pure vanilla extract or vanilla bean paste

1/8 teaspoon of salt

1/3 cup of erythritol

2 cups of canned coconut milk, full fat

Directions

Stir together the vanilla extract, salt, sweetener and milk.

If you don't have an ice cream machine, freeze the mixture in ice cube trays then use a high speed blender to blend the frozen cubes or thaw them enough to blend in a regular blender or food processor.

If you have an ice cream machine, just churn according to the manufacturer's directions

Eat as it is or freeze for a firmer texture

Nutritional info per serving: Calories 184, Proteins 1.8g, Carbs 4.4g and Fats 19.1g

Low Carb Dairy Free Fondue

Prep time: 0 minutes

Cook time: 5 minutes

Total time: 5 minutes

Yields: 4 servings

Ingredients

¼ to ½ cup of canned coconut milk, full fat

2 oz. 100% cocoa dark chocolate

1 teaspoon of vanilla extract

Tiny pinch of salt

Liquid stevia to taste

Directions

Microwave directions:

Place everything apart from the stevia in a microwave safe bowl and microwave for 30 seconds. Remove and stir until glossy and smooth.

Add the additional coconut milk, as you desire then if the mixture is still hard, microwave in 10 second increments while stirring in between until it is smooth without any lumps. Add in the stevia slowly, a few drops at a time to your desired sweetness

Stove directions:

In a small saucepan, heat the coconut milk on low heat until warmed throughout and smooth. Add in all the other ingredients apart from the Stevia.

Keep stirring frequently until the chocolate completely melts and the mixture becomes glossy and smooth. Add in more coconut milk if the mixture is too thick for your taste

Remove mixture from heat and slowly add in the stevia a little at a time until you achieve your desired sweetness. Serve with some berries.

Nutritional info: Calories 102.1, Proteins 2.1g, Carbs 4.9g and Fats 10.2g

Keto Chocolate Truffle

Prep time: 10 minutes

Cook time: 20 minutes

Total time: 30 minutes

Yields: 15 truffles

Ingredients

¼ cup cocoa powder

¼ teaspoon kosher salt

1 teaspoon vanilla extract

1 medium avocado, mashed

1 cup of dark chocolate chips, melted

Directions

Combine the melted chocolate with the salt, avocado and vanilla in a medium bowl.

Stir the ingredients until fully combined and smooth. Place in the refrigerator for 15 to 20 minutes to firm up slightly.

Once the chocolate mixture has stiffened, use a small spoon or a small cookie scoop to scoop approximately 1 tablespoon of the chocolate mixture.

Roll the chocolate in the palm of your hand to a round shape then roll in the cocoa powder.

Nutritional info per serving: Calories 90, Proteins 2g, Carbs 3.2g and Fats 3g

Chocolate Hazelnut Cookies

Prep time: 5 minutes

Cook time: 5 minutes

Total time: 10 minutes

Yields: 20 cookies

Ingredients

1 cup of crushed hazelnuts

½ cup of sticky sweetener of your choice

2 cups of chocolate hazelnut spread of your choice

¾ cup of coconut flour

1 tablespoon of liquid of your choice

Directions

Prepare a large plate by lining with parchment paper then set aside.

Add all your ingredients to a large mixing bowl and mix very well to form dough. Add liquid of your choice if the batter is too thick.

Add the crushed hazelnuts to a small mixing bowl. Roll the dough into small balls using your hands then roll each of the balls into the bowl with the crushed hazelnuts.

Place the hazelnut-coated balls onto the lined plate and press each into a cookie shape. Refrigerate until firm.

Drizzle with melted chocolate if desired.

Nutritional info per cookie: Calories 103, Proteins 4.5g, Carbs 4.5g and Fats 7.5g

Chocolate Blueberry Clusters

Prep time: 25 minutes

Cook time: 0 minutes

Total time: 25 minutes

Yields: 15 blueberry clusters

Ingredients

2 cups of blueberries

1 tablespoons of coconut oil

1 ½ cups of melted, semi-sweet chocolate chips

Flaky sea salt for garnish

Directions

Prepare a small baking sheet by lining it with parchment paper.

Mix the coconut oil with the melted chocolate in a medium bowl.

Scoop a small dollop of the chocolate mixture and pour on the parchment then top with 4 to 5 blueberries

Drizzle chocolate on top of the blueberries and sprinkle with the flaky sea salt

Freeze for 10 minutes until set

Serve.

Nutritional info per serving: Calories 70, Proteins 2g, Carbs 2g and Fats 4.5g

Avocado Chocolate Mousse

Prep time: 5 minutes

Cook time: 0 minutes

Total time: 5 minutes

Yields: 2 servings

Ingredients

1/8 teaspoon of salt

¼ to ½ cup of coconut milk

½ cup of cocoa powder or chocolate chips

1 teaspoon of pure vanilla extract

Flesh of 2 ripe avocados (240 grams)

Pinch of stevia or 2 to 6 tablespoons of sweetener of your choice

Directions

If you are using the chocolate chips, melt them carefully before you begin.

For both versions, combine all the ingredients in a food processor or blender and process until completely smooth.

For a thicker mousse use less milk and for a creamier/thinner result use more milk. If using the chocolate chips use only a pinch of stevia or 2 to 3 tablespoons of the sweetener of your choice. If you are using the cocoa powder, use a higher amount of sweetener

If you don't have a food processor or a blender you can try mashing the ingredients together, however, it will not be nearly as smooth.

Nutritional info per serving: Calories 103, Proteins 4g, Carbs 5g and Fats 7.5g

Strawberry Cheesecake Salad

Prep time: 15 minutes

Cook time: 0 minutes

Total time: 15 minutes

Yields: 4 servings

Ingredients

¼ cup of almond flour

8 oz. of fresh strawberries chopped and hulled

2 tablespoons of sugar free syrup

10 grams of freeze dried strawberries, in powder form

½ cup of heavy cream

8 oz. of cream cheese

Directions

Place half the heavy cream and the cream cheese in a stand mixer bowl and mix on slow until ingredients are fully combined.

Add the remaining heavy cream and mix again. Add the syrup and the freeze dried strawberry powder and mix until fully combined

Add the almond flour and the fresh strawberries and stir using your hand until fully mixed

Pour mixture into a serving dish and refrigerate as desired

Nutritional info per serving: Calories 363, Proteins 5g, Carbs 9g and Fats 34g

Keto Snacks and Smoothies

Prep time: 5 minutes

Cook time: 8 minutes

Total time: 13 minutes

Yields: 8 bites

Ingredients

2 basil leaves or a little more as you need

1 tomato, large

4 oz. mozzarella

1 eggplant aubergine, medium/small

Good quality olive oil

Directions

Cut off the eggplant end then cut it into thin slices of around 0.25cm/0.1 inch thick lengthwise. Do away with the smaller pieces that are mostly skin and not as long as the other pieces. Slice the tomato and the mozzarella as well and cut the basil leaves thinly.

Heat a griddle pan and brush the eggplant slices lightly with olive oil. Alternatively, you can drizzle on the olive oil and rub over quickly before it gets absorbed.

Place the oiled eggplant slices on the earlier warmed pan and grill for a few minutes on each side until they have light grill marks and soften. Before the second side is completely done, add a bigger piece of mozzarella cheese in the thicker part of the eggplant slice.

Top with a slice of tomato then add a smaller piece of mozzarella to the thinner end of the eggplant. Sprinkle the top with basil and a little ground pepper if you wish. Leave it to cook for one more minute then remove it carefully from the pan – a little liquid will come out from the cheese and the tomato so let it drain off.

Roll the eggplant from the thin end, which has only the cheese. It probably will not roll completely so once it is close; hold it together using a cocktail stick.

For the best taste, serve warm but you can also serve at room temperature.

Nutritional info per serving: Calories 59, Protein 3g, Carbs 3g and Fats 3g

Parmesan Cauliflower Steak

Prep time: 5 minutes

Cook time: 25 minutes

Total time: 30 minutes

Yields: 4 servings

Ingredients

¼ cup parmesan cheese

4 tablespoons of butter

1 large head cauliflower

2 tablespoons of roasted garlic seasoning blend

Pepper and salt to taste

Directions

Preheat your oven to 400 degrees F. Remove the cauliflower leaves.

Place butter in microwave to melt then mix with the seasoning blend to make a paste.

Brush the cauliflower steaks with the butter mixture then season with pepper and salt for taste

Place a non-stick pan over medium heat and cook the steaks until lightly browned for around 2-3 minutes. Carefully flip the steaks to cook the other side.

Place the browned steaks on a lined baking sheet then place in oven and allow to cook until tender and golden for 15-20 minutes.

Sprinkle parmesan cheese on top and serve.

Nutritional info per serving: Calories 90, Proteins 5g, Carbs 4g and Fats 4g

Garlic Baked Brie Recipe

Prep time: 2 minutes

Cook time: 20 minutes

Total time: 22 minutes

Yields: 2 servings

Ingredients

3-4 garlic cloves, diced

7 ounces brie

4-6 sage leaves or any herb of your choice

Directions

Preheat your oven to 350 degrees F or 180 degrees C.

Place the brie in an oven friendly dish then score the top. Fill the holes with diced garlic and top with sage leaves or any other herb you love.

Place into the earlier preheated oven for around 15 to 20 minutes or until cooked to your liking

You can serve as it is or with cucumber or celery.

Nutritional info per serving: Calories 40, Proteins 1g, Carbs 2g and Fats 2g

Baked Cheddar Parmesan Crisps

Prep time: 5 minutes

Cook time: 7 minutes

Total time: 12 minutes

Yields: 4 servings

Ingredients

¾ cup of cheddar cheese, shredded

¾ cup of parmesan cheese, shredded

Optional:

1 teaspoon of Italian seasoning

Directions

Preheat your oven to 400 degrees F (204 degrees c).

Use parchment paper to line a large baking sheet

Place the cheeses in a small bowl and stir.

Pour uniform tablespoon sized amounts of the combined cheeses onto the baking sheet, 5 cm (2 inches) apart – leave enough room because the cheeses will spread. If you are using Italian seasoning, sprinkle it over the top.

Place the sheet in the oven and bake until the edges begin to brown for around 6 to 8 minutes – keep a close eye on them as they go from done to burned pretty fast.

Leave the cheese chips in the pan to cool lightly then transfer to paper towels to get crispy and drain.

Nutritional info: Calories 152, Protein 11g, Carbs 1g and Fats 11g

Creamed Leeks with Garlic and Cream Cheese

Prep time: 5 minutes

Cook time: 10 minutes

Total time: 15 minutes

Yields: 2 servings

Ingredients

25g of cream cheese

2 cloves of garlic, crushed

2 tablespoons of butter

2 large leeks, sliced

Black pepper

Directions

Heat the butter in a large saucepan and cook the garlic.

Add the sliced leeks and leave to cook until soft, stirring throughout.

Remove saucepan from heat and stir in the black pepper and cream cheese

Nutritional info per serving: Calories 105, Protein1.2g, Carbs 6.4g and Fats 8.4g

Creamy Mushroom and Cauliflower Risotto

Prep time: 1 minute

Cook time: 5 minutes

Total time: 6 minutes

Yields: 2 servings

Ingredients

1 cup sliced mushrooms

2 garlic cloves, sliced

1 head Cauliflower

Coconut oil or butter for frying

¼ to ½ cups of liquid (water, milk, vegetable stock or cream)

Optional: Parmesan for topping

Directions

Rice the cauliflower with a grater box or in a food processor.

Heat a little butter or coconut oil in a frying pan over medium to high heat, and then add the mushrooms and garlic once hot and sauté until reduced.

Add the liquid of your choice and the cauliflower and simmer gently until the cauliflower is cooked through, ensuring you stir regularly.

Transfer to a bowl and top with parmesan cheese if desired

Nutritional info per serving: Calories 100, Proteins 1g, Carbs 2g and Fats 8g

Arugula Strawberry Salad

Prep time: 10 minutes

Cook time: 10 minutes

Total time: 20 minutes

Yields: 2 servings

Ingredients

¼ cup of sliced almonds, roasted lightly

6 organic strawberries, quartered

4 cups of baby arugula

Lemon vinaigrette:

2 tablespoons of avocado oil

2 tablespoons of lemon juice

Sea salt and pepper (freshly ground)

Directions

Place the almonds, strawberries and arugula on a plate.

For the lemon vinaigrette, whisk together the avocado oil, lemon juice, pepper and salt.

Drizzle the vinaigrette over the salad and use the rest of the dressing on the side.

Finish by sprinkling additional fresh ground pepper and salt to taste.

Nutritional info per serving: Calories 228, Protein 4g, Carbs 7g and Fats 21g

Creamy Keto Smoothie

Prep time: 5 minutes

Cook time: 0 minutes

Total time: 5 minutes

Yields: 1 serving

Ingredients

¼ cup of plain or vanilla whey protein

1 tablespoon of ground chia seeds

½ teaspoon of cinnamon

1 tablespoon of extra virgin coconut oil or MCT oil

½ cup of coconut milk (4 fl oz. /120 ml)

½ cup of water and a few ice cubes

Directions

Add the ground chia seeds, cinnamon, protein powder and coconut milk in a blender. Add the ice and if desired a few drops of Stevia. Blend ingredients until smooth and serve immediately

* If you use coconut oil, ensure you blend well because it solidifies - MCT oil is more suitable in making cold drinks because it does not solidify

Nutritional info: Calories 467, Protein 23.6g, Carbs 8.2g and Fats 40.3g

Coconut Vanilla Smoothie

Prep time: 1 minute

Cook time: 0 minutes

Total time: 1 minutes

Yields: 1 serving

Ingredients

3 ounces of frozen organic sweet cherries

1/8 teaspoon of pure vanilla powder

3 1/3 ounces of filtered water

2 ½ ounces of full fat canned coconut milk

7 to 8 ice cubes

Pinch of finely ground sea salt

Directions

Add the full fat coconut milk, filtered water, vanilla powder, sea salt, frozen organic sweet cherries and ice cubes in that order to the blender and process until smooth

Enjoy

Nutritional info per serving: Calories 400, Protein 20.2g, Carbs 8g and Fats 16g

Low Carb Strawberry Smoothie

Prep time: 1 minute

Cook time: 0 minutes

Total time: 1 minute

Yields: 1 serving

Ingredients

2 tablespoons of almond

½ teaspoon of cinnamon

½ cup of frozen organic strawberries

1 cup of unsweetened vanilla almond milk

Optional:

1 tablespoon of chia seeds

Directions

Place all the ingredients in a blender or magic bullet and blend until smooth.

Nutritional info: Calories 100, Protein 3g, Carbs 8g and fats 1g

Chocolate Coconut Smoothie

Prep time: 2 minutes

Cook time: 0 minutes

Total time: 2 minutes

Yields: 1 serving

Ingredients

1/4 teaspoon of turmeric

1/2 cup shredded unsweetened coconut

1/2 ripe avocado

1/4 cup of cacao powder

1 can of full fat coconut milk

1 cup frozen cherries

A few ice cubes and filtered water

Directions

Place all ingredients except the ice and water in your blender of choice.

Add the ice and water required to fill the blender to the top fill line and blend to your desired consistency

*You can decrease the avocado by half and add a cup of greens for increased nutrient boost

Nutritional info per serving: Calories 120, Proteins 20g, Carbs 5g and Fats 30g

Coconut Bacon

Prep time: 5 minutes

Cook time: 25 minutes

Total time: 30 minutes

Yields: 2 servings

Ingredients

1 tablespoon of monk fruit

1 tablespoon of soy sauce or Braggs liquid aminos

2 tablespoons of liquid smoke

3 ½ cups of flaked coconut, unsweetened

1 tablespoon of water

Optional:

1 teaspoon of smoked paprika

Directions

Pre heat your oven to 325 degrees F.

In a large mixing bowl, combine the water, maple syrup, Braggs and liquid smoke.

Toss the flaked coconut into the liquid mixture. If using smoked paprika, add then toss to coat the coconut evenly

Pour the coconut mixture into a non-stick baking sheet.

Bake for 20-25 minutes flipping the "bacon" around every 5 minutes using a spatula so that it cooks evenly. If you don't keep an eye on the "bacon" and flip it regularly, it will definitely burn, so please do.

If you make more than you can eat and you want to store the rest, place in a sealed container or bag and refrigerate for up to a month

Nutritional info per serving: Calories 200, Protein 13g, Carbs 20g and Fats 23g

Lemon & Garlic Sautéed Brussels sprouts

Prep time: 0 minutes

Cook time: 10 minutes approx.

Total time: 10 minutes

Yields: 2 servings

Ingredients

Juice of ½ a lemon

Zest of 1 lemon

1 lb. /500g of Brussels sprouts, halved

3 to 4 cloves of garlic, peeled and diced

Coconut oil or butter for frying

Salt and pepper to taste

Optional: parmesan

Directions

Heat the coconut oil or butter in a frying pan. Add the garlic once hot and cook until fragrant.

Add the pepper, salt and the halved Brussels sprouts and cook until browned and softened.

Add the lemon juice and lemon zest and cook to your liking.

Serve as it is or top with parmesan or any other cheese of your choice

Nutritional info per serving: Calories 40, Proteins 2g, Carbs 1g and Fats 7g

Stuffed Baby Peppers

Prep time: 10 minutes

Cook time: 10 minutes

Total time: 20 minutes

Yields: 4 servings

Ingredients

Cream cheese, full fat

Baby peppers

Optional: herbs

Directions

Wash each baby pepper thoroughly and slice off the top. Scoop out the little seeds inside.

Using a blunt knife such as butter knife, stuff each pepper slowly with cream cheese until they are completely filled.

*You can store in the fridge for up to 3 days.

Note: You can vary the stuffed baby peppers by adding flavors to the cream cheese such as sliced celery, chili flakes, jalapenos, pepperoni pieces, sun-dried tomatoes etc.

Nutritional info per serving: Calories 40, Proteins 1g, Carbs 1g and Fats 8g

Keto Kale Chips

Prep time: 5 minutes

Cook time: 20 minutes

Total time: 25 minutes

Yields: 2 servings

Ingredients

1 teaspoon of curry powder

1 tablespoon of olive oil

100 grams of kale

Salt to taste

Directions

Wash the kale thoroughly and dry. Separate the kale leaves from the stalk then chop into small chip-sized pieces. Mix with the olive oil, curry powder and salt

Bake at 150 degrees C on a wire rack until crispy for about 20 minutes.

Serve immediately as they will not stay crisp for long.

Nutritional info per serving: Calories 88, Proteins 2g, Carbs 5g and Fats 7g

Creamy Cucumber Salad

Prep time 5 minutes

Cook time: 0 minutes

Total time: 5 minutes

Yields: 2 servings

Ingredients

2 tablespoons of lemon juice

2 tablespoons of mayo

1 cucumber, sliced then quartered

Freshly ground pepper and salt to taste

Instructions

In a small bowl, mix the lemon juice, mayo and cucumber slices. Add pepper and salt to taste. Serve.

Nutritional info per serving: Calories 116, Protein 1g, Carbs 2g and Fats 12g

Avocado Salad

Prep time: 5 minutes

Cook time: 0 minutes

Total time: 5 minutes

Yields: 1 cup

Ingredients

1 tablespoon of balsamic vinegar

1 tablespoon of extra virgin oil

1 ripe avocado

Salt to taste

Directions

Cut the ripe avocado in half. Remove the pit then using a small knife score each half into cubes. Scoop out the avocado using a spoon

Toss with balsamic vinegar, extra virgin oil and salt

Nutritional info per serving: Calories 50, Proteins 1g, Carbs 2g and Fats 3g

Avocado, Almond & Blueberry Salad

Prep time: 1 minute

Cook time: 0 minutes

Total time: 1 minute

Yields: 1 serving

Ingredients

1-2 tablespoons Trader Joes Green Goddess Dressing

1/2 ripe avocado

1 oz of Blueberries

15g of sliced almonds

1/2 cup Trader Joes Cruciferous Crunch

1 cup of Arugula Mix

Optional: 1 tablespoon of MCT oil

Directions

Combine all ingredients

Recipe note

If you are not eating immediately, place the MCT oil and the dressing on the side

Nutritional info per serving: Calories 256.4, Proteins 6.2g, Carbs 16.5g and Fats 20.2g

Brussels Sprouts Caesar Salad

Prep time: 5 minutes

Cook time: 0 minutes

Total time: 5 minutes

Yields: 4 servings

Ingredients

1/4 cup of Parmesan cheese, freshly shaved

1/2 teaspoon of black pepper

1/2 teaspoon of kosher salt

1/3 cup of olive oil

1 large lemon

1 pound of fresh Brussels sprouts shredded

Directions

Juice and zest the lemon then whisk with the olive oil, pepper and salt

Toss with the freshly shaved parmesan cheese and Brussels sprouts

Serve.

Nutritional info per serving: Calories 233, Proteins 6g, Carbs 10g and Fats 19g

Feta Lemon Coleslaw

Prep time: 1 minute

Cook time: 1 minute

Total time: 2 minutes

Yields: 2-4 servings

Ingredients

2 spring onions, finely chopped

1/2 cup of Feta cheese, crumbled

1/2 head white cabbage, finely sliced

3 tablespoons of Olive oil

Juice of ½ lemon

1/2 teaspoon of salt

1/2 teaspoon of black pepper

Directions

Place the green onions and the white cabbage in a bowl.

Blend the olive oil, lemon and feta cheese in another bowl then add the pepper and salt

Pour over the cabbage and toss until coated.

Enjoy

Nutritional info per serving: Calories 165, Proteins 4g, Carbs 5g and Fats 14g

Lemon & Feta Summer Zucchini Salad

Prep time: 10 minutes

Cook time: 0 minutes

Total time: 10 minutes

Yields: 6 servings

Ingredients

1.5 oz. of lemon juice

1.5 oz. of olive oil

1/2 cup of feta cheese

1/4 cup of grape tomatoes, halved

2 large zucchini, spiraled

1/2 teaspoon of salt

Optional: 1 teaspoon of fresh oregano, chopped

Directions

Place the oregano, feta cheese, tomatoes and zucchini in a medium bowl.

Stir together the lemon juice, salt and olive oil in another bowl.

Pour the dressing over the salad and serve.

Nutritional info per serving: Calories 109, Proteins 2g, Carbs 3g and Fats 9g

Tofu Fries

Prep time: 10 minutes

Cook time: 10 minutes (if you cook in 2 batches)

Total time: 20 minutes

Yields: 2 servings

Ingredients

3 tablespoons of parsley

18 oz. tofu

Olive oil

Salt and pepper

Directions

Remove the tofu from the package and cut into ½-inch slices.

Use paper towels to blot them dry then slice lengthwise again into half strips.

Gently place the tofu strips onto a double layer of paper towels then add another double layer of paper towels on top and press down lightly.

Allow the tofu strips to rest for around 5 minutes then season with pepper and salt.

Heat about 3 inches of oil in a large fryer or pot to 350 degrees F

Lay the tofu strips onto the hot oil in small batches so that the fries don't touch each other as they might stick together. Cook until golden brown for about 3-4 minutes.

Remove the tofu fries from oil. Remove the excess oil by blotting on paper towels

Nutritional info per serving: Calories 145, Proteins 16g, Carbs 4g and Fats 9g

Tempeh Stir-Fry

Prep time: 5 minutes

Cook time: 15 minutes

Total time: 20 minutes

Yields: 3 servings

Ingredients

2 tablespoons of coconut oil divided

227 grams of tempeh cut into ½ inch cubes

1 tablespoon of sesame seeds for serving

3 tablespoons of coconut aminos

1 teaspoon of ginger root, minced

3 cloves of garlic, minced

1 tablespoon of avocado

Directions

Optional: Steam the tempeh. Wrap the tempeh in a wet paper towel then place in a microwave safe bowl and microwave in 2 minutes increments for a total of 4 to 6 minutes – stop and let the tempeh sit for a minute or 2 between the increments.

In a small bowl, stir together the ginger, garlic and the coconut aminos.

Use a tablespoon of oil to coat the bottom of a large skillet then place over medium heat.

Add the tempeh cubes in just a single layer and cook until browned on multiple sides for about 10 minutes flipping once or twice

Remove from heat then sprinkle with the sesame seeds. Serve and enjoy

Nutritional info per serving: Calories 289, Proteins 14.9g, Carbs 13.2g and Fats 19.6g

Keto Smoked Maple Tempeh

Prep time: 5 minutes

Cook time: 25 minutes

Total time: 30 minutes

Yields: 3 servings

Ingredients

1 tablespoon of olive oil

1 tablespoon of low sodium tamari

2 tablespoons of sugar free maple syrup

8oz. block of tempeh

¼ to ½ teaspoon of smoked salt

Directions

Preheat your oven to 350 degrees F then line your baking sheet with parchment paper.

In a small mixing bowl, whisk together the tamari, sugar free syrup, salt and olive oil and let this to sit for a few minutes in order for the flavors to melt together and the salt to dissolve.

Slice the tempeh into ¼-inch thick pieces then dip into the maple mixture. Ensure the tempeh is completely covered then place onto the baking sheet. Repeat this procedure for each slice.

Pour or brush the remaining sauce over the tempeh then place the baking tray in the preheated oven.

Bake for around 25 minutes, optionally flipping halfway through

Nutritional info per serving: Calories 195, Proteins 15.8g, Carbs 3.4g and Fats 12.7g

Tempeh Hash Browns

Prep time: 2 minutes

Cook time: 5 minutes

Total time: 7 minutes

Yields: 1 serving

Ingredients

8 oz. / 1 pack of light life flax tempeh

Oil for frying – depends on your cooking equipment; the tempeh should be completely immersed

Salt to taste

Directions

Based on your hash brown preference either grate or slice the tempeh and deep fry until it is caramel brown.

Remove from the oil and blot using paper towels to remove excess oil.

Salt generously.

Nutritional info per serving: Calories 427, Proteins 40g, Carbs 24g and Fats 18.7g

Spinach Almond Stir-Fry

Prep time: 0 minutes

Cook time: 10minutes

Total time: 10 minutes

Yields: 2 servings

Ingredients

1 tablespoon of coconut oil for cooking

3 tablespoons of almond slices

1 lb. of spinach leaves

Salt to taste

Directions

Add the coconut oil into a large pot and place over medium heat.

Add the spinach and allow it to cook down.

Add the salt to taste once the spinach is cooked down and stir.

Stir in the almond slices before serving.

Nutritional info per serving: Calories 150, Proteins 8g, Carbs 4g and Fats 11g

Green Spinach Smoothie

Prep time: 5 minutes

Cook time: 0 minutes

Total time: 5 minutes

Yields: 1 serving

Ingredients

1 scoop of amazing grass greens powder

1 cup of unsweetened coconut milk (from refrigerated cartons not cans)

2 Brazil nuts

10 raw almonds

2 cups of spinach or kale

Optional: tablespoon of potato starch, scoop of whey protein and a tablespoon of psyllium husks or psyllium seeds

Directions

Place the coconut milk, Brazil nuts, almonds and spinach into the blender first and blend until pureed.

Add the remaining ingredients and blend well

Nutritional info per serving: Calories 380, Proteins 12g, Carbs 13g and Fats 30g

Conclusion

We have come to the end of the book. Thank you for reading and congratulations for reading until the end.

If you found the book valuable, can you recommend it to others? One way to do that is to post a review on Amazon.

Don't forget to leave a review for this book on Amazon!

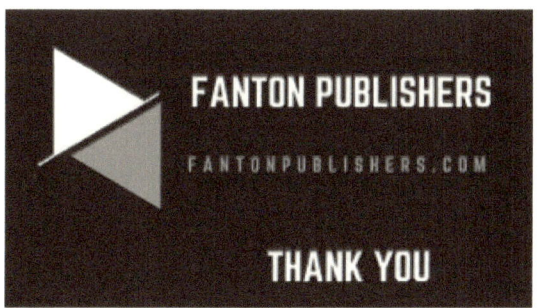

Do You Like My Book & Approach To Publishing?

If you like my writing and style and would love the ease of learning literally everything you can get your hands on from Fantonpublishers.com, I'd really need you to do me either of the following favors.

1: First, I'd Love It If You Leave a Review of This Book on Amazon.

2: Check Out My Other Keto Diet Books

KETOGENIC DIET: Keto Diet Made Easy: Beginners Guide on How to Burn Fat Fast With the Keto Diet (Including 100+ Recipes That You Can Prepare Within 20 Minutes)- New Edition

KETOGENIC DIET: Ketogenic Diet Recipes That You Can Prepare Using 7 Ingredients and Less in Less Than 30 Minutes

Ketogenic Diet: With A Sustainable Twist: Lose Weight Rapidly With Ketogenic Diet Recipes You Can Make Within 25 Minutes

Ketogenic Diet: Keto Diet Breakfast Recipes

Fat Bombs: Keto Fat Bombs: 50+ Savory and Sweet Ketogenic Diet Fat Bombs That You MUST Prepare Before Any Other!

[Snacks: Keto Diet Snacks: 50+ Savory and Sweet Ketogenic Diet Snacks That You MUST Prepare Before Any Other!](#)

[Desserts: Keto Diet Desserts: 50+ Savory and Sweet Ketogenic Diet Desserts That You MUST Prepare Before Any Other!](#)

[Ketogenic Diet: Ketogenic Diet Lunch and Dinner Recipes](#)

[Ketogenic Diet: Keto Diet Cookbook For Vegetarians](#)

[Ketogenic Diet: Ketogenic Slow Cooker Cookbook: Keto Slow Cooker Recipes That You Can Prepare Using 7 Ingredients Or Less](#)

Note: This list may not represent all my Keto diet books. You can check the full list by visiting my [Author Central](#): amazon.com/author/fantonpublishers or my website http://www.fantonpublishers.com

Get updates when we publish any book on the Ketogenic diet: http://bit.ly/2fantonpubketo

Closely related to the keto diet is intermittent fasting. I also publish books on Intermittent Fasting.

One of the books is shown below:

[Intermittent Fasting: A Complete Beginners Guide to Intermittent Fasting For Weight Loss, Increased Energy, and A Healthy Life](#)

Get updates when we publish any book on intermittent fasting: http://bit.ly/2fantonbooksIF

To get a list of all my other books, please fantonwriters.com, my author central or let me send you the list by requesting them below: http://bit.ly/2fantonpubnewbooks

3: Let's Get In Touch

Antony

Website: http://www.fantonpublishers.com/

Email: Support@fantonpublishers.com

Twitter: https://twitter.com/FantonPublisher

Facebook Page: https://www.facebook.com/Fantonpublisher/

My Ketogenic Diet Books Page: https://www.facebook.com/pg/Fast-Keto-Meals-336338180266944

Private Facebook Group For Readers: https://www.facebook.com/groups/FantonPublishers/

Pinterest: https://www.pinterest.com/fantonpublisher/

4: Grab Some Freebies On Your Way Out; Giving Is Receiving, Right?

I gave you 2 freebies at the start of the book, one on general life transformation and one about the Ketogenic diet. Grab them here if you didn't grab them earlier.

Ketogenic Diet Freebie: http://bit.ly/2fantonpubketo

5 Pillar Life Transformation Checklist: http://bit.ly/2fantonfreebie

5: Suggest Topics That You'd Love Me To Cover To Increase Your Knowledge Bank

I am looking forward to seeing your suggestions and insights; you could even suggest improvements to this book. Simply send me a message on Support@fantonpublishers.com.

PSS: Let Me Also Help You Save Some Money!

If you are a heavy reader, have you considered subscribing to Kindle Unlimited? You can read this and millions of other books for just $9.99 a month)! You can check it out by searching for Kindle Unlimited on Amazon!

www.ingramcontent.com/pod-product-compliance
Lightning Source LLC
Chambersburg PA
CBHW030156100526
44592CB00009B/307